Strength Training for Men:

How To Build Muscle, Boost Power, and Transform Your Physique

By

Jeffrey Davison

Table of Contents

Chapter 1: Introduction to Strength Training for Men

Strength training stands out as a fundamental pillar of physical well-being in a society where health and fitness are of utmost importance. The significant advantages and concepts of strength training are explained to men in this chapter, setting the platform for a life-changing path toward improved strength, muscle growth, and general vigor.

Strength Training's Power

Strength training helps you develop resilience, increase your self-confidence, and embrace the potential of your own body in addition to growing muscle. This section outlines the numerous effects of strength training on your mental and emotional health in addition to your physical health. The advantages are extensive and significant, ranging from better posture and higher bone density to heightened metabolism and improved physical performance.

The Benefits of Strength Training for Fitness and General Health

There are few efforts that can compare to the value of including strength training in your regimen in the quest for a better and more satisfying life. Strength training has a wealth of advantages that improve your general well-being in addition to aesthetics and bodybuilding. In-depth discussion of the tremendous value of strength training is provided in this chapter, along with examples of how it can benefit all aspects of your quest for fitness and health.

A Solid Base for Practical Living

Strength training is about preparing your body for the demands of daily living, not just about gaining muscle for show. Resistance training builds muscle strength, which directly translates into increased functional capacity.

Your capacity to carry out daily duties effectively and with a lower risk of injury is improved by having a stronger body, which helps you move heavy objects and climb stairs with ease.

Management of Metabolism and Weight

The powerful impact strength training has on metabolism is one of the sport's unsung heroes. Muscles burn calories even when at rest since they are metabolically active tissues. Strength training regularly helps you gain lean muscle mass, which raises your resting metabolic rate. As you expend more calories during the day and find it simpler to acquire and maintain a healthy body composition, this can have a substantial impact on weight management.

Bone Longevity and Health

As we age, keeping strong bones becomes increasingly important for avoiding age-related diseases like osteoporosis. Strength training workouts that involve weight bearing promote bone development and mineral density. By consistently putting resistance on your bones, you lower the chance of fractures and improve your mobility and quality of life over the long run.

Improvement of Cardiovascular Health

Strength training has benefits for your cardiovascular system in addition to the world of weights and resistance. Your heart rate can be raised and your cardiovascular endurance improved by performing circuit-style strength exercises with short rest periods. Strength and cardiovascular exercise have the added advantage of being time-effective ways to increase general fitness and heart health.

Managing Hormones for Mental Health

Hormone control is positively impacted by strength exercise. It encourages the release of endorphins, or "feel-good" hormones, which lessen the signs of anxiety and depression and relieve stress. Strength exercise can also have a good effect on testosterone levels, which are important for muscular growth and general health.

Injury Reduction and Prevention

An effective strength training program can serve as a barrier against accidents. Increasing the stability and support around your joints lowers your risk of strains, sprains, and other ailments. Strength training can also be extremely important for injury recovery, assisting you in regaining strength and mobility following periods of immobilization or physical treatment.

Myths and Fallacies Regarding Strength Training

Strength training is not an exception to the many myths and misconceptions that exist in the fitness and exercise world. In order to embrace the full potential and advantages of strength training, these myths must be dispelled. This chapter clarifies frequent misunderstandings, giving you the knowledge and perspective you need to approach strength training with accuracy and assurance.

Myth: Using weights causes you to gain weight.

The notion that strength training invariably results in a bulky body is one of the most popular misunderstandings about it. In actuality, a number of variables, such as hormone levels, food, workout intensity, and genetics, affect how much muscle you can actually gain.

Strength training should not result in excessive muscle growth in women in particular because their hormonal makeup restricts muscle growth in comparison to men. Strength training frequently produces a toned, lean physique as opposed to one that is bulky.

Myth: Only young people should do strength training

Another myth is that strength training is only appropriate for young, athletic people. In actuality, strength training has advantages for people of all ages, from youth to the elderly.

Through concentrated strength training, older persons can, in particular, see improvements in bone density, balance, and functional mobility. Strength training is adaptable to different fitness levels and life phases, therefore age should never be a barrier to participation.

Myth: Cardio Is Better for Weight Loss Than Strength Training

Although it is true that cardiovascular activity burns calories, the notion that it is preferable to strength training for weight loss is a misconception.

As previously established, strength training increases muscle mass, and muscle is a metabolically active tissue that consumes calories even while at rest. Exercises that combine cardiovascular activity with strength training have a synergistic impact that quickens weight loss and enhances general fitness.

Myth: Strength training puts you at risk of being hurt.

While there are risks associated with every form of exercise, proper strength training done with the right form and technique does not carry these risks. In fact, one of the best methods to avoid injuries is through strength training.

Strains, sprains, and other injuries that may occur from regular activity can be prevented by strengthening muscles and stabilizing joints. Under the direction of an experienced trainer, learning and using good form can significantly reduce any risks.

Myth: Strength training can help you lose fat in specific areas.

It's a prevalent misperception that specialized activities will help you lose weight in particular body parts. For instance, performing a ton of crunches won't instantly reduce abdominal fat.

Systematic fat loss happens all across the body and is impacted by things like heredity and total calorie balance. Strength training boosts metabolism, which aids in fat loss, but spot-reduction is still a myth. Effective fat loss requires a combination of a balanced diet and all-encompassing, full-body strength training.

No Pain, No Gain is a myth.
The saying "no pain, no gain" has led many people astray by leading them to believe that exercise must be difficult in order to be effective. Pain is not a sign of improvement, even though challenging workouts can cause some discomfort.

Pain may be a sign of improper form, overuse, or a hidden injury. Gains are much more easily sustained and successful with proper programming, moderate progression, and attentive listening to your body's cues.

Differences between strength training and other forms of exercise

Different exercise forms cater to differing goals and outcomes in the vast world of physical fitness. Strength training stands out among them as a different discipline with its own special qualities and advantages.

This chapter explains how strength training differs from other forms of exercise and explains how it benefits physical growth, improved health, and general well-being.

Concentrate on Building Muscle and Strength

As the name suggests, the main focus of strength training is increasing muscle strength and endurance. Strength training focuses on specific muscle groups rather than the heart and lungs, which are primarily targeted by cardiovascular activities. Strength training promotes muscle fibers to adapt and grow through regulated resistance and weight-bearing movements, leading to an improvement in strength and muscular definition.

Engagement and Adaptation of Muscle Fibers

Depending on the intensity and kind of the activity, strength training uses both fast-twitch and slow-twitch muscle fibers. While slow-twitch fibers are involved in endurance, fast-twitch fibers are in charge of power and explosive motions.

Strength training fosters a well-rounded muscular growth that improves both strength and endurance capabilities by focusing on both types of fibers.

Growth Through Progressive Overload

Progressive overload is one of the pillars of strength training. In this idea, the resistance or weight used in exercises is gradually increased over time.

Strength training encourages continual adaptation and growth by routinely pushing the muscles beyond their initial limit. Strength training differs from other activities that might not emphasize increasing overload thanks to this methodical approach.

Rest and Recuperation for Best Results

Rest and recovery are acknowledged as essential elements of the process in strength training. After being subjected to resistance, muscles need time to recover and get stronger.

Between strength training sessions, there should be enough time for rest to give muscles time to heal and adapt. In contrast to some high-intensity exercises that necessitate longer recovery times, this planned strategy.

Localized and practical advantages

While strength training benefits particular muscle groups locally, cardiovascular exercise benefits general cardiovascular health. This makes it ideal for focusing on specific areas that need work.

Strength training also improves functional fitness, which makes it easier for you to carry out daily duties. The improved muscle stability and strength make lifting, carrying, and even keeping posture easier.

Multiple Modalities and Flexibility

From bodyweight exercises, resistance bands, and even functional training, strength training offers a wide variety of methods. Strength training is now available to people of all fitness levels, preferences, and constraints because to its versatility.

Strength training's adaptability enables personalization and scalability, unlike some routines that could be more specialized.

Within the field of exercise, strength training is recognized as a dynamic and narrowly focused discipline. It differs from other forms of physical activity due to its focus on muscle development, progressive overload, targeted adaptation, and functional improvement.

Whether your objectives involve boosting strength, enhancing endurance, or developing a balanced and robust physique, you are better positioned to harness its transforming power by recognizing the special characteristics of strength training.

Chapter 2: Setting Your Goals and Creating a Plan

Setting specific objectives and creating a well-thought-out plan are crucial first steps in starting an effective strength training program. In order to ensure that your efforts produce the best results and long-lasting success, this chapter explores the value of clearly identifying your objectives and developing a personalized strategy that is in line with your desires.

The Influence of Setting Goals

Clarifying your goals before beginning any project is essential. Setting goals gives you direction, inspiration, and a point of reference for gauging your success in the world of strength training.

It doesn't matter if your objective is to gain more muscle mass, improve functional strength, or reach particular fitness milestones;

having a clear vision of what you want to do will help you focus your efforts.

Setting SMART Objectives

SMART objectives are clear, quantifiable, attainable, pertinent, and time-bound. This framework makes sure that your objectives are clear and doable.

SMART goals offer clarity and a road map for success, so aim for specifics like "increase bench press weight by 20% in three months" or "complete a full pull-up within six weeks" rather than generic aims like "get fit" or "get stronger."

Considering Your Position

It's essential to evaluate your present level of fitness in order to develop a useful plan. This assessment offers a starting point from which you may monitor your development.

This evaluation may include calculating your one-rep maximum for important exercises, checking your flexibility, and noting any physical limits. You can use this information to set reasonable goals and to guide your training strategy.

Developing Your Training Program

It's time to create a training program that is specifically suited to your goals after you've determined your objectives and evaluated your starting place.

Exercise selection, frequency, intensity, and progression should all be part of your plan. You may choose to do full-body workouts or split routines that target separate muscle groups on different days, depending on your degree of skill and preferences.

Overloading Progressively and Periodization

The notion of progressive overload, which calls for gradually increasing resistance and intensity to promote muscular growth, is central to your training program.

Periodization, a planned method for handling different training factors, is included to guarantee consistency while avoiding plateaus. Periodization may involve switching up the rep ranges between exercises and switching between high- and low-intensity phases.

Dietary intake and healing

A good strength training program includes activities outside of the gym. The right diet and recovery techniques are essential to attaining your objectives. Protein, carbs, and healthy fats should all be consumed in sufficient amounts to support muscle growth and recovery. To avoid overtraining and advance general wellbeing, it's equally important to prioritize sleep, manage stress, and incorporate rest days.

Monitoring and Modifying

Monitoring your progress frequently is crucial for assessing how well your plan is working. Maintain a workout diary to note your workouts, sets, reps, and weights so you can track your progress over time. Do not be afraid to make changes if you discover stalls or departures from your objectives. Your plan will continue to be in line with your changing needs if your approach is flexible.

Setting objectives and coming up with a detailed strategy are essential components of a fruitful strength training journey. You are prepared to start down a route that is both rewarding and successful by setting SMART goals, figuring out where you are starting from, creating a tailored training schedule, and combining sensible diet and recuperation techniques. Keep in mind that your plan is not set in stone; routine review and modification guarantee that your path through strength training is dynamic and in line with your goals.

1. Choosing your fitness objectives: increasing strength overall or gaining muscle mass
Prior to starting a strength training program, it's important to identify your precise fitness objectives. Your training efforts are guided by these goals, which also influence your routines, diet, and general strategy.

This chapter digs into three main fitness objectives: building muscle, losing body fat, and improving overall strength. It examines the intricacies of each objective and offers guidance to help you make an informed decision.

2. Gaining Muscle: Discovering Your Inner Sculptor

Your main objective should be to focus on muscle gain if you want to build a more muscular physique. Resistance exercise and specialized nutrition are used during this journey to promote muscular hypertrophy, which is the process of expanding the size of muscle fibers.

Compound motions and isolation exercises will both be incorporated into your training program, which will be focused on activities that promote muscular growth. Your dietary plan will involve eating more calories than you need, with an emphasis on getting enough protein to support tissue growth and repair.

3. Carving Out Your Definition for Weight Loss

The objective of fat reduction is to reduce extra body fat while maintaining muscle mass. In order to accomplish this, you must spend more energy than you take in. Strength training must be a part of your regimen if you want to keep muscle while decreasing fat.

Your metabolism can be increased and fat loss can be accelerated by compound motions that use several muscle groups. High-intensity interval training (HIIT), which increases calorie burn, can further support your efforts.

4. Increasing General Strength: Laying a Resilient Foundation

Your goal is to develop physical versatility if your main objective is to improve your overall strength and functional fitness. Compound exercises that simulate everyday motions like squats, deadlifts, and overhead presses will be prioritized in your training program.

Your ability to lift heavier weights and your performance in these fundamental exercises will be the main goals. Your capacity to complete daily duties and take part in a variety of physical activities is improved by achieving this aim.

5. Making a Decision: Considerations and Crossroads

It's crucial to match your decision with your preferences, way of life, and level of fitness as you weigh the many fitness goals. Choose the path that aligns with your goals because each one calls for a different approach to training and diet. Remember that you can switch between these objectives based on your shifting priorities; they are not mutually exclusive.

6. Adapting Your Approach: Making It Personal is Important

Customization is crucial no matter what your fitness objective is. Your results will depend on things like your genetics, metabolism, and unique response to exercise. You can create a strategy that meets your specific needs and goals by seeking the advice of trainers or fitness industry professionals. Additionally, it's important to practice patience and consistency because results don't happen overnight.

The beginning of any strength training adventure is defining your fitness objectives, whether they be to increase overall strength, lose fat, or develop muscle.

You can create the conditions for a meaningful and successful journey by comprehending the nuances of each objective and selecting the one that most closely aligns with your desires.

Your journey should be marked by progress, perseverance, and a dedication to obtaining the outcomes that are consistent with your vision of a healthier, stronger you. Keep in mind that your goals may change over time.

Setting realistic expectations and evaluating your current level of fitness

It's important to accurately assess your present fitness level and set reasonable goals for your growth before starting a strength training program. This chapter explores the value of self-evaluation and the relevance of creating realistic goals to make sure your route to strength and fitness is both efficient and long-lasting.

1. The Benefits of Self-Evaluation

Your fitness journey starts with a self-evaluation. It gives you a quick overview of your physical attributes, including your strengths and potential growth areas. You can customize your training program by undertaking an honest and unbiased evaluation to better understand your strengths and weaknesses.

2. Physical Evaluations

Physical evaluations include a variety of measurements and examinations that enable you to determine your starting point. These evaluations may involve measurements of important body dimensions, analyses of body composition, flexibility tests, and simple strength tests. By recording these starting points, you may follow your development and observe observable advancements over time.

3. Fitness Evaluations

Evaluation of your degree of fitness is important in addition to physical measurements. You can evaluate your present skills by doing tests like the push-up challenge, plank hold time, and flexibility evaluations.

These standards give you a base from which to grow and develop.

4. Having reasonable expectations

The next step after determining your present level of fitness is to set reasonable goals for your advancement. Being passionate and motivated is normal, but it's also crucial to maintain perspective. Setting realistic goals helps avoid later frustration and disappointment.

5. Recognizing the Journey

Understand that the road to strength and fitness is not a straight one. Cycles of rapid improvement followed by plateaus are signs of progression. With perseverance and adaptation, plateaus can be surmounted. They are a normal part of the process. Understanding this ebb and flow enables you to keep the big picture in mind.

6. Progress-Influencing Factors

Your growth is affected by a number of variables, including genetics, lifestyle, nutrition, sleep, stress, and consistency. Although you have no influence over all of these factors, you may make the best use of them to aid in your travels.

You have influence over how consistently you train and how well you recuperate, and these factors have a big impact on your outcomes.

7. Celebrate achievements and minor victories.

Celebrate the tiny triumphs along the road as you progress toward your bigger objectives. These accomplishments, like raising your lifting ability, enhancing your endurance, or setting a new personal record, are signs of development. Taking note of these victories and appreciating them helps you stay motivated and committed.

Setting reasonable expectations and evaluating your current level of fitness are essential first stages in your strength training journey. You can lay up a plan for success by being aware of where you are right now and setting attainable goals.

Keep in mind that growth takes time, and that consistency of effort, adaptation, and patience are the keys to long-term success. Keep your goals in mind as you negotiate the difficulties and victories, and take pleasure in the changes that happen as you progress toward strength and wellbeing.

creating a customized strength training program based on your objectives
A critical step toward achieving the best results is developing a customized strength training program that is in line with your unique goals.

Explores the nuances of creating a customized program while taking your fitness goals, experience level, time constraints, and preferences into account. You'll travel through your strength training trip with direction and effectiveness if you have a well-crafted plan.

1. Establishing Your Goals

Establish your fitness objectives explicitly before creating your plan. Do you want to boost your general strength, lose weight, gain muscle, or all of the above? Your exercise choice, training volume, and intensity will be determined by your objectives.

2. How to Evaluate Your Experience Level

Your experience level affects the complexity and advancement of your program, regardless of whether you are a beginner, intermediate, or advanced learner. While experts might include advanced techniques and higher loads, beginners might begin with basic workouts and less weights.

3. Selecting Exercises

Choose workouts that help you achieve your goals. Squats, deadlifts, bench presses, and overhead presses are examples of compound exercises that are essential for increasing overall strength and muscular mass. Specific muscle groups might be the focus of isolation exercises for additional definition or rehabilitation needs.

4. Choosing the Training Frequency

The design of your program is heavily influenced by how frequently you train each week. Beginners would benefit from three to four sessions each week, which would provide enough time for recovery. More seasoned athletes may work out more frequently or use split regimens to concentrate on different muscle groups on separate days.

5. Organizing Your Exercises

Your workouts can be organized in a variety of ways, such as with full-body routines, upper/lower splits, or muscle-specific days. To target various muscle groups, each workout should include a mix of complex and isolation exercises. Plan for enough recuperation time in between sets to support intensity maintenance.

6. Rep ranges and Progressive Overload

The cornerstone of strength training continues to be progressive overload. To promote muscular growth and strength gains, gradually increase the resistance or weight you are lifting. Goal-specific repetition ranges include lower reps (about 1-6), moderate reps (around 8-12), and high reps (15+) that promote muscular endurance.

7.. Integration of nutrition and recovery

Incorporate a nutrition plan that supports your goals with your strength training program. Make sure you consume enough protein and are in a modest calorie excess for muscle growth. Create a calorie deficit while keeping your protein intake steady for fat loss. Put recuperation first by taking care of your sleep, water, and stress.

8. Changing and Moving Forward

Reevaluate your strategy frequently to gauge progress and make changes. To avoid plateaus, increase weights, adapt routines, or change rep ranges. To gradually test your muscles in new ways, gradually include advanced techniques like supersets, drop sets, and pyramid sets.

9. Tracking and recording

To keep track of your exercises, weights, reps, and sets, keep a training notebook. With the aid of this paperwork, you can keep track of your progress, spot trends, and decide with confidence how beneficial your training program is.

10. Consultation with Experts

If hesitant, think about speaking with a personal trainer or fitness expert. Their knowledge may assist you in customizing your plan to meet your objectives, preferences, and constraints, assuring you are on the right route.

It takes careful evaluation of your goals, experience, and unique characteristics to create a customized strength training program. With a well-designed program in place, you'll start down a path of development, expansion, and empowerment.

Your body and your abilities will change as you stick to your plan, make adjustments as necessary, and remain dedicated, getting you closer to the level of strength and fitness you desire.

Chapter 3: Essential Strength Training Exercises

Key exercises that target significant muscle groups, advance functional fitness, and establish the framework for dramatic effects comprise the basis of strength training. The fundamental strength training exercises that make up the bulk of your workout regimen are covered in this chapter. These exercises not only increase strength and muscular growth, but they also improve everyday functioning and general agility.

1. Squats

The quadriceps, hamstrings, glutes, and calves are among the lower body muscles that the squat targets. It is a basic complex action. The core is also activated for stability. The goblet squat, front squat, and other variations enable you to change the weight and concentrate on other muscle areas.

2. Deadlifts

The best exercise for gaining strength and useful power is the deadlift. They work the muscles of the posterior chain, such as the glutes, hamstrings, and traps, as well as the lower back. A variety of deadlift variants, including conventional, sumo, and Romanian deadlifts, are available to target different muscle regions and accommodate diverse body types.

3. Table Press

The bench press is a well-known exercise for the upper body that predominantly works the pectoralis major, as well as the shoulders and triceps. It is a crucial exercise for increasing upper body muscular growth and strength.

4. Vertical Press

The overhead press, sometimes referred to as the shoulder press, works the triceps, upper back, and shoulder deltoid muscles. This exercise helps to create a more balanced physique by strengthening the upper body and stabilizing the shoulders.

5. Rows

The upper back muscles, especially the lats, rhomboids, and rear deltoids, are the focus of rowing workouts like bent-over rows and seated rows. Rowing helps build the entire upper body, strengthen the back, and improve posture.

6. Pull-Ups/Chin-Ups

These bodyweight workouts put stress on the shoulders, biceps, and upper back. While chin-ups provide more emphasis on the biceps, pull-ups primarily target the back muscles. Additionally, the grip power and upper body balance are improved by these workouts.

7. Push-Ups

The chest, shoulders, and triceps are worked out with the adaptable bodyweight exercise known as the push-up. They may be adjusted to accommodate individuals with varying levels of fitness, making them a practical tool for enhancing upper body strength and muscular endurance.

8. Lunges

Exercises that isolate the quadriceps, hamstrings, glutes, and calves include lunges. They increase balance, stability, and lower body strength. Your routine will be more interesting with variations including forward, backward, and lateral lunges.

9. Planks

For core stability and engagement, planks are crucial. They exercise the deep abdominal muscles that support your spine and help to maintain general postural strength, including the rectus abdominis, obliques, and transverse abdominis.

10. Hip sways

Hip thrusts work the core while also focusing on the glutes and hamstrings. This exercise is very good for developing glutes that are firm and defined.

A thorough strength program is built on including these fundamental strength training exercises in your regimen. These exercises create the foundation for attaining your fitness objectives and developing a strong, robust body by working the key muscle groups, enhancing functional fitness, and encouraging balanced growth. As you include these exercises into your strength training program, keep in mind to focus perfect technique, increasing loading, and consistency.

Breakdown of Basic Compound Exercises: Strength and Power Building

Strength training's cornerstone is compound exercises since they work several muscle groups and effectively grow muscles. The most important compound exercises will be broken down in this chapter, along with information on how to do them, how your muscles will be activated, and what they can accomplish for your strength-training goals.

1. The foundation of lower body strength is the squat

Exercises for the lower body's classic quadriceps, hamstrings, glutes, and lower back include squats. Stand with your feet shoulder-width apart, your chest high, and your back straight to complete a squat. While keeping your knees in alignment with your toes, lower your hips back and down. In order to go back to the beginning position, drive through your heels. Squats promote mobility and core stability in addition to strengthening the legs.

2. Total-Body Powerhouse: Deadlifts

The capacity to increase strength and power across the entire body is unmatched by anything else. They concentrate on the forearms, glutes, hamstrings, and lower back muscles. Start by standing with a barbell in front of you and your feet hip-width apart. To take an overhand or mixed grip on the bar, stoop at the hips and knees. Maintaining a neutral spine, stretch your hips and knees to lift the bar. Grip strength, posture, and lifting capability are all enhanced by deadlifts.

3. Bench Press: Power and Muscle in the Upper Body

The pectorals, deltoids, and triceps are the main muscle groups that the bench press predominantly targets in the upper body. Lay on a bench, take a little wider-than-shoulder-width hold on the barbell, and bring it to your chest.

Reposition the bar so that it is at the beginning point. Incline, decline, and dumbbell bench presses are examples of bench press variants. This exercise encourages the development of balanced muscles while improving upper body strength.

4. Shoulder and upper body strength with the overhead press

The overhead press, sometimes referred to as the shoulder press, works the triceps, upper back, and shoulder deltoid muscles. Press a barbell or dumbbells above while standing with your feet shoulder-width apart.

Press the weight back up after lowering it to shoulder height. This exercise helps to create a more balanced physique by strengthening the upper body and stabilizing the shoulders.

5. Rows: Upper Body Muscular Balance and the Back

Rows are essential for working the muscles of the upper back, such as the lats, rhomboids, and rear deltoids. Rows can be performed sitting or bent-over. Hinging at the hips while maintaining your back straight, row a barbell or dumbbells toward your lower ribs to do bent-over rows. Rows help to build the entire upper body, strengthen the back, and improve posture.

6. Upper Body Strength and Grip for Pull-Ups and Chin-Ups

Bodyweight workouts that work the upper back, biceps, and shoulders include pull-ups and chin-ups.

Pull your body upward until your chin clears the bar by grasping a bar with palms facing away (pull-up) or toward you (chin-up) and pulling. Additionally, the grip power and upper body balance are improved by these workouts.

7. Push-Ups: A Flexible Upper Body Exercise

The chest, shoulders, and triceps are worked out with the adaptable bodyweight exercise known as the push-up. Start in a plank posture, squat down to the floor, and then push yourself back up.

Since push-ups can be altered to accommodate various levels of fitness, anybody may use them to develop upper body strength and muscular endurance.

A powerful, well-balanced body is attained by mastering basic compound exercises. Each of these exercises works many different muscle groups, encourages functional strength, and advances overall athleticism.

These exercises should be a part of your routine whether you're a novice or a seasoned lifter since they serve as the cornerstone of a successful strength training regimen.

Compound exercises have a transforming effect in increasing strength, power, and muscle growth as you work to improve your form, add resistance, and advance over time.

Suitable posture, technique, and typical errors to avoid

Strength training places a premium on performing movements with good form and technique. This chapter emphasizes the need of keeping proper form during exercises, offers instructions for each one, and lists frequent errors to avoid. The efficiency of your workouts will be maximized and the danger of injury is reduced by placing a high priority on good technique.

Proper Form and Technique for squatting
1. Keep your toes turned slightly outward and your feet shoulder-width apart.
2. Pushing your hips back and maintaining your back straight while doing so will start the action.
3. Keeping your spine neutral, lower your hips until your thighs are parallel to the floor.
4. To get back up, drive your heels into the floor.

Common Errors:
1. Allowing the inward fall of your knees.
2. stooping too low or arching your back.
3. not diving deep enough or diving too low.

Proper Form and Technique for Deadlifts

1. Grasp the barbell with your hands slightly outside of your knees as you stand with your feet hip-width apart.
2. To lower your torso and maintain your back flat, hinge at your hips and knees.
3. By extending your hips and knees, you may lift the bar while keeping it close to your body.
4. Stand tall and with a neutral spine, extending your hips fully.

Common Errors:

1. Especially towards the bottom of the action, rounding your back.
2. Starting the exercise with your hips too high or low will result in injury.
3. not utilizing your legs or your core sufficiently.

Proper Form and Technique for the Bench Press

1. Your eyes should be pointed at the barbell while you lay on the bench.
2. Straighten your wrists while taking a slightly broader than shoulder-width grip on the barbell.
3. Maintaining a 45-degree angle with your elbows, lower the bar to your chest.
4. Reposition the bar to its initial position by pressing it.

Common Errors:

1. Extending your back too far.
2. Either flaring your elbows or bouncing the bar off your chest.
3. Too broad or too narrow of a grip on the bar.

Proper Form and Technique for the Overhead Press

1. Place the barbell in your hands just outside your shoulders while standing with your feet shoulder-width apart.
2. While maintaining your core engaged, stretch your arms and press the bar above.
3. Avoid slouching or overextending your lower back while you press.
4. Controlled bar lowering to shoulder level.

Common Errors:

1. Extending your lower back while performing the press.
2. Getting moving with your lower body.
3. Unnecessarily letting your elbows stretch out.

Proper Form and Technique for Rows

1. While maintaining a straight back, hinge at the hips while you hold the barbell or dumbbells in your hands.
2. Squeezing together your shoulder blades, lift the weight toward your lower ribs.
3. Fully extend the weight while lowering it under control.

Common Errors:

1. Start the exercise from your lower back.
2. using your neck to pull or hunching your shoulders forward.
3. attempting to lift the weight with excessive force.

Proper Form and Technique for Performing Pull-Ups and Chin-Ups

1. When performing a pull-up or chin-up, grip the bar with your hands facing away from you.
2. Engage your core while hanging from the bar with your arms straight.
3. Till your chin clears the bar, lift your body up while starting from the chest.
4. Controlled body lowering will result in a dead hang.

Common Errors:

1. using considerable momentum or swinging.
2. without extending your arms all the way at the bottom.
3. raising your shoulders toward your ears while shrugging.

Proper Form and Technique for Push Ups

1. Start off with your hands slightly wider than shoulder width in a plank stance.
2. By bending your elbows while maintaining a 45-degree angle, lower your body.
3. Reposition your body to the beginning position by pushing.

Common Errors:

1. letting your hips lift or sag.
2. putting your hands too far or too close together.
3. not walking with a straight back and heels.

In strength training, proper form and technique must be used at all times. You may improve the safety and efficacy of your exercises by adhering to these rules and avoiding frequent blunders. By consistently using proper form, you may guarantee that you're not only protecting yourself from harm but also effectively hitting the targeted muscle areas. Always remember that getting advice from an experienced trainer will help you improve your technique and get a more in-depth understanding of your form.

The significance of measuring your progress and avoiding progressive overload

The essential concepts that generate persistent growth and success in strength training are progressive overload and measuring your progress. This chapter explains the significance of these ideas, how they advance your fitness goals, and how to use them to their fullest potential.

Progress via Progressive Overload

To increase muscular development and strength gains over time, progressive overload includes gradually increasing the demands placed on your muscles. To continue noticing benefits when your muscles adjust to a certain load, you must challenge them with progressively larger weights, more resistance, or increased intensity. The efficacy of strength training is built on this idea.

Progressive Overload Advantages
Increased muscular mass and definition: These are the results of your muscles having to adapt and grow as a result of being overloaded.

Gains in Strength: By persistently pushing your physical boundaries, you increase your strength and functional potential.

Gaining muscle mass increases your resting metabolic rate, which promotes fat loss and helps you maintain a healthy weight.

Injury Prevention: Gradual progression reduces the chance of overuse injuries since it gives your body time to adjust to heavier loads.

Prevention of Plateaus: When your muscles are no longer being used, stagnation can happen. Continuous improvement is ensured via progressive overload.

Progressive Overload Techniques: Increasing Weight: As you get stronger, gradually increase the weight of your lifts.

Reps and Sets: Increase the quantity of reps and sets you do with a certain weight.
Increasing Intensity: To raise intensity, shorten rest periods, use drop sets, or employ complex exercises.

Exercise Variation: Change up your routine to attack your muscles from various angles and to give them new challenges.

Monitoring Your Development: The Road to Improvement

Tracking your development is essential to effective strength training. It offers unbiased information that enables you to assess your performance, make wise modifications, and maintain motivation throughout your trip.

Gains from Monitoring Your Progress

1. **Results that are Measurable:** You can clearly notice increases in strength, endurance, and muscular development.

2. **Motivation:** Seeing a rise in your stats and making progress motivates you to continue.

3. **Goal Achievement:** Tracking enables you to keep focused on your objectives and, if necessary, change your strategy.

4. **Identification of Plateaus:** You can identify when progress slows down and make the required adjustments by examining trends.

5. **Form and Technique Improvement:** By watching how you perform, you may improve your form and technique.

Techniques for Monitoring Your Progress

1. Keep track of the exercises, sets, repetitions, and weights used during each session in a workout journal.

2. Use digital applications to track your exercises and measure your development over time.

3. Measure important body components and take regular images to document any observable changes.

4. Track performance data, such as your one-rep maximum (1RM), for important exercises to determine progress.

A successful strength training program must include progressive loading and progress monitoring. You build a road plan for continual improvement by methodically tracking your performance and gradually pushing your muscles. With the help of these concepts, you can modify your exercises, establish and meet objectives, and enjoy the transforming effects of strength training as you grow into a stronger, healthier, and more competent version of yourself.

Chapter 4: Creating Effective Workouts

Creating successful exercises requires a combination of science, strategy, and personal objectives. This chapter explores the subtleties of designing exercises that support your goals, push your body, and guarantee steady growth. You'll be able to design workouts that optimize your strength training trip if you comprehend the fundamentals of workout structure, activity choice, and training variables.

Exercise Design and Elements

Warm-up: To stimulate blood flow, raise your heart rate, and get your muscles and joints ready for the activities ahead, start each workout with a vigorous warm-up.

Exercises that target particular muscle groups, such as complex and isolation moves, make up your main workout. Selecting exercises, deciding on sets and repetitions, and scheduling rest periods are all parts of structuring your primary workout.

Cool Down: Spend time cooling down with static stretches to improve flexibility, encourage healing, and lessen pain after exercise.

Compound Movements: A Balanced Approach to Exercise Selection Compound workouts that work many muscle groups should take precedence. These exercises, which include squats, deadlifts, bench presses, rows, and overhead presses, serve as the building blocks of your workout.

Isolation Movements: To target specific muscles, combine complex workouts with isolation movements. These include tricep extensions, leg curls, and calf lifts, in addition to bicep curls.

Training Variables: Customizing Volume and Intensity

Choose rep ranges for your sets based on your objectives. Lower repetitions (1-6) put the emphasis on strength, medium repetitions (8–12) on muscular growth, and higher repetitions (15+) on endurance.

Adjust the weight or resistance you use in each exercise to change the intensity so that you are gradually overloading your muscles.

Rest Intervals: The length of the breaks in between sets affects how intense and concentrated your workouts are. While shorter rest periods increase muscular endurance, longer rest periods enable the return of maximum strength.

Full-body exercises and split routines

Divide your workouts into several sessions to focus on various muscle groups on different days. Upper/lower, push/pull, and body component splits are typical splits.

Exercises for the Whole Body: Perform complex exercises that work many muscle groups at once. For novices or those who have a limited amount of time, full-body exercises are effective.

Advancement and Adaptation

Linear Progression: To promote muscle growth and strength improvements, gradually increase weights over time.

Periodization: Use periodization to change your training volume and intensity, avoiding plateaus and maximizing your growth.

Monitoring and Assessment

Maintain a workout journal to keep track of the exercises, sets, repetitions, and weights you utilize throughout each session.

Measure your one-rep maximum (1RM) for the main exercises to determine your progress.

Changing Workouts: Make regular adjustments to your workouts based on your performance, goals, and input from your body.

Effective workout design necessitates careful consideration of structure, activity choice, training factors, and adaptability. You may create routines that support your goals, test your body, and put progressive overload first, which will pave the way for continuous development and change.

Remember that each workout is an opportunity to advance, improve your strength, and get closer to attaining your fitness goals as you put the lessons from this chapter into practice.

Combining flexibility, cardio, and strength training

Strength training is only one component of a well-rounded fitness plan. Optimizing overall health, performance, and well-being requires a balance between strength training, aerobic activity, and flexibility work. We'll examine the advantages of each element in this chapter and provide tips for finding a healthy balance in your workout program.

What Is Strength Training Used For?

Muscle hypertrophy, strength, and functional ability are the main goals of strength training. It encourages bone density, increases metabolism, and helps contour the body. Strength training serves as the cornerstone of your fitness journey, regardless of your objectives, which may include muscle building, fat loss, or enhanced sports performance.

Cardiovascular exercise's advantages

Cardio, also known as cardiovascular exercise, enhances endurance, lung capacity, and cardiovascular health. It increases general fitness while burning calories and assisting with weight management. Regular cardio exercise, such as jogging, cycling, swimming, or high-intensity interval training (HIIT), improves recovery and complements strength training by fostering cardiovascular efficiency.

The Value of Flexibility in the Workplace

Yoga, static stretching, and other forms of flexibility practice improve posture, increase joint mobility, and lower the risk of injury. Additionally, it promotes relaxation and muscular repair. By including flexibility exercises in your program, you may prevent the muscular tightness that comes from strength training and help maintain total body balance.

Techniques for Balance

1. Prioritize your objectives: Decide on your main fitness goals, such as muscular growth, cardiovascular health improvement, or flexibility improvement. Spend more attention on the component that supports your core objective.

Create a weekly schedule with strength training, cardio workouts, and flexibility work.

2. Design a balanced routine: As advised by health standards, strive to do at least 150 minutes of moderate-intensity cardio or 75 minutes of vigorous-intensity cardio per week.

3. On alternate days: Separate your strength training and cardio workouts to give your muscles and cardiovascular system enough time to heal.

4. Combine Modalities: Use interval or circuit training that combines cardio and strength training for a time-effective method to work on both in a single session.

5. Include flexibility: After your workouts or on rest days, set aside time for flexibility exercises. Flexibility, balance, and relaxation can all be improved by yoga exercises or sessions.

6. Pay Attention to Your Body's Signals: Listen to your body. Prioritize recuperation and flexibility work if you're feeling exhausted or stressed to avoid burnout and lower your risk of injury.

7. Schedule Active Rest Days: To keep your body moving without overexerting it, schedule active rest days that include low-intensity exercises like walking, swimming, or light yoga.

The secret to a thorough fitness regimen that improves all facets of your well-being is to balance strength training with cardio and flexibility exercises. By judiciously combining these elements, you may develop a physique that is strong, flexible, and competent, in addition to reaching your fitness objectives.

Keep in mind that maintaining balance is dynamic and that your priorities and habits may change as you go. Enjoy the advantages of a well-rounded approach to health and vitality by accepting the variety of your fitness path.

Include procedures for warm-ups, cool-downs, and recovery.

Effective strength training programs include adequate warm-ups, deliberate cool-downs, and proactive recovery techniques in addition to the actual workout. The importance of warm-ups, cool-downs, and recovery practices in maximizing your strength training journey and fostering long-term wellbeing is examined in this chapter.

Warm-Ups: Getting Your Body Ready for Movement

Warm-ups are essential to get your body ready for exercise, boost blood flow to the muscles, and improve joint mobility. A proper warm-up may reduce the risk of injury, enhance performance, and emotionally get you ready for the workouts ahead.

Dynamic Stretches: Carry out dynamic stretches that resemble the motions you'll make when working out. Examples of dynamic warm-up activities include hip rotations, arm circles, and leg swings.

Cardiovascular Activity: To gradually raise your heart rate and warm up your muscles, engage in light aerobic activities like running, cycling, or brisk walking.

Exercises for improving joint range of motion include mobility drills. The health of your joints will benefit from shoulder rotations, hip hinges, and ankle circles.

Cool-Downs: Reducing Intensity by Easing Your Body Out

Your body may gradually shift from a high-intensity workout to a resting condition by using cool-downs. This can lessen muscular pain, minimize dizziness, and improve circulation for faster healing.

Perform static stretches: Stretches that concentrate on the main muscle groups. To increase flexibility and relieve stress, hold each stretch for 15 to 30 seconds.

Light Cardio: To gradually reduce your heart rate and bring your body into a state of relaxation, engage in light aerobic activity like strolling.

Self-massage with a foam roller: This might help you loosen up knotted muscles. This promotes muscle healing and lessens discomfort in the muscles.

Techniques for Recuperation: Aiding Your Body's Repair

Techniques for proactive recuperation aid in muscle healing, lower the likelihood of overuse injuries, and enhance total training effectiveness. Utilizing these techniques will enable you to recover from each session stronger.

Rest Days: Set aside days for total rest or low-intensity exercise to allow your muscles and central nervous system to heal.

Nutrition and Hydration: To refill your energy reserves and promote muscle recovery, eat a balanced diet and drink enough water.

Prioritize getting enough sleep to assist in the creation of hormones, muscle repair, and general wellbeing.

Active recuperation: To encourage blood flow and recuperation without overexertion, take part in low-intensity activities like yoga, swimming, or light strolling on your rest days.

Regular massages or self-myofascial release with a foam roller help alleviate tension in the muscles and speed up tissue repair.

Your total performance and wellbeing depend on including warm-ups, cool-downs, and recovery exercises in your strength training program. These techniques lay the groundwork for injury avoidance, improved performance, and speedy recuperation, enabling you to constantly pursue your fitness objectives with tenacity and zeal.

Accept these factors as essential parts of your fitness journey and develop an all-encompassing strategy that prioritizes the planning, execution, and recuperation stages of your exercises.

Chapter 5: Nutrition for Strength and Muscle Gain

More than simply weightlifting is necessary to develop your strength and muscle; you also need a solid dietary strategy to complement your workout. In order to help you get the best results, this chapter goes deeply into the fundamentals of nutrition for strength and muscle building. It provides information on macronutrients, meal planning, and supplements.

The Nutritional Foundation; Macronutrients

Protein: Protein is necessary for the development and repair of muscles. Aim for a diet high in protein, including foods like tofu and tempeh as well as lean meats, chicken, fish, eggs, dairy products, and legumes.

Carbohydrates: Carbohydrates sustain muscular glycogen reserves and provide you with the energy you need to get through your workouts. Instead of simple carbs, choose complex ones from whole grains, fruits, vegetables, and legumes.

Fats: Good fats contribute to the generation of hormones and general health. Include foods like avocados, almonds, seeds, olive oil, and oily salmon in your diet.

Timing your meals to support your training

Pre-Workout Nutrition: To offer sustained energy and promote muscular function, eat a balanced breakfast with carbs and protein around 1-2 hours before your workout.

Post-Workout Nutrition: Within 30 to 60 minutes of your workout, consume a protein-rich meal or smoothie. Your muscles are most capable of absorbing nutrients and recovering during this time.

Meal Frequency: To ensure a consistent supply of nutrients for muscle growth and repair, aim for frequent meals and snacks throughout the day.

Caloric Intake: Energy Balance

Caloric Surplus: You must be in a caloric surplus—consuming more calories than you burn off—in order to gain muscle. Put an emphasis on calorie-rich, nutrient-dense meals.

Follow your weight, measurements, and strength increases to see how you're doing. Based on your accomplishments and goals, modify your calorie intake.

Hydration: Commonly Ignored Yet Essential for Performance

Water: Drink enough water throughout the day. Dehydration can delay muscle recovery and reduce performance.

Electrolytes: Replace any electrolytes lost via perspiration, particularly during strenuous exercise. Eat or drink things that are high in electrolytes.

Taking Supplements to Improve Your Nutrition

Whey, casein, and plant-based protein powders can all help you achieve your protein requirements, particularly when it's difficult to get enough from complete meals.

Creatine: By raising intramuscular energy levels, creatine monohydrate supplementation improves strength and muscle growth.

Branched-chain amino acids (BCAAs) may be helpful during periods of rigorous exercise because they assist muscle repair.

Your quest for strength and muscular building depends heavily on your diet. You may maximize your body's capacity to respond to your training efforts by being aware of the significance of macronutrients, meal planning, calorie intake, hydration, and supplements.

You can efficiently feed your body, promote muscle growth, and develop the strength and physique you want by creating a dietary plan that supports your training program and is in line with your goals. Always maintain consistency in your exercise and eating to achieve long-term results.

Tips for meal preparation and supplements for the best outcomes

The use of supplements and meal preparation can greatly improve your progress with strength training. You can intentionally promote muscle development, enhance recovery, and maximize your performance by carefully supplying your body with the proper foods and supplements. This chapter offers helpful advice on nutrition and food planning to help you get the most out of your strength training.

Planning your meals for strength training

1. Put protein first: Include a high-quality protein source in each meal to help muscle development and repair. Lean meats, poultry, fish, eggs, dairy products, legumes, and plant-based protein sources are a few examples.

2. Consume complex carbs: to maintain energy levels throughout exercise and replace glycogen storage. Excellent sources include whole grains, fruits, vegetables, and legumes.

3. Healthy Fats: Include healthy fats in your diet to promote hormone production and general wellness. Healthy food options include avocados, almonds, seeds, olive oil, and fatty seafood.

4. Consistent Meal Frequency: To provide a consistent supply of nutrients and energy for training and recuperation, aim for frequent meals and snacks throughout the day.

5. Nutrition Prioritize protein and carbs before and after your workout to fuel your session and aid in recuperation. To improve muscle recovery, eat a protein-rich meal or shake right after working out.

6. Hydration: Make sure you get enough water throughout the day to stay hydrated. Dehydration can have a detrimental effect on performance and strength.

Adding Supplements to Strength Training

1. Protein supplements: If getting enough protein from whole foods is difficult, you might want to try whey, casein, or plant-based protein supplements. These can be practical choices for after a workout or while you're on the run.

2. Creatine: One of the most extensively studied supplements, creatine monohydrate has been demonstrated to increase muscular growth, strength, and power. For best outcomes, consume it prior to or following exercise.

3. Branched-Chain Amino Acids (BCAAs): During strenuous training sessions or when you're in a calorie deficit, BCAAs can help with muscle rehabilitation and prevent muscle breakdown.

4. Omega-3 Fatty Acids: Fish oil-based omega-3 supplements, which are frequently used to enhance joint health and reduce inflammation, can hasten the healing process.

5. Multivitamins and Minerals: A high-quality multivitamin will help fill any nutrient gaps in your diet and make sure you're getting all the vitamins and minerals you need for optimum performance and recovery.

6. Scheduling and dose: Consider scheduling depending on your particular demands and training plan while adhering to supplement dose recommendations.

7. Whole Foods First: Supplements should enhance, not replace, a healthy diet. Give whole foods first priority as your main source of nutrition.

Individualization and advice

The specific dietary requirements of each person depend on their age, gender, aspirations, and metabolism. To develop a customized food plan and supplement regimen that suits your unique needs and preferences, speak with a licensed dietitian or nutritionist. With this knowledge, you may adjust your strategy for the best possible strength training outcomes.

Planning your meals and using supplements will help you achieve the best results from your strength training. You create the conditions for dramatic success by mindfully combining supplements that match your nutritional requirements and strategically planning your meals to fuel your workouts, improve recovery, and encourage muscle growth.

To reap the rewards and reach your best potential in your strength training adventure, keep in mind that consistency in your nutritional practices and supplement usage is essential.

Chapter 6: Rest and Recovery Strategies

The continuous quest for improvement in the world of fitness and sports sometimes obscures a crucial component of training: rest and recuperation. Allowing your body enough time to rest and recuperate is crucial to getting the most out of your fitness journey, even if it may seem paradoxical.

In this thorough book, we'll examine the science of rest and recovery, discuss their importance, and offer a variety of practical tips to help you make the most of these sometimes overlooked components.

Understanding rest and recovery science

Whether you're a top athlete, a weekend warrior, or just trying to live a healthy lifestyle, rest and recovery are essential parts of any training program. Understanding how your body reacts to exercise and stress is crucial to understanding the relevance of these ideas.

1. Stress and Adaptation: Physical

Your body is stressed when you exercise, especially when you perform demanding activities like strength training. Your muscle fibers suffer tiny damage as a result of this stress, which sets off an adaptive reaction called supercompensation.

The injured muscle fibers are essentially rebuilt by your body, making them stronger and more resilient than before. Rest, however, is important since this adaptive process takes time and resources.

2. Exhaustion and Overtraining

Overtraining, a condition in which the body is continually under stress without enough time to recuperate, can result from not getting enough sleep.

Overtraining may lead to diminished performance, on-going weariness, a higher chance of injury, and even mental burnout. To avoid slipping into this harmful condition, proper rest and recuperation are crucial.

The Value of Recovery and Rest

1. Muscle Repair and Growth: The body fixes the small muscle damage brought on by exercise when we are at rest. Muscle development and enhanced strength result from this mending process.

2. Hormonal Balance: Getting enough sleep helps to maintain hormonal equilibrium, which includes the production of growth hormone, testosterone, and cortisol. These hormones are essential for muscle development, repair, and stress management.

3. Mental Health: Exercise can have a negative impact on one's mental health. Your mind can heal with rest, which lowers your risk of burnout, elevates your mood, and sharpens your attention.

4. Better Performance: Adequate rest makes sure that your body is emotionally and physically ready for the upcoming session. Over time, this results in higher performance and outcomes.

Effective Strategies for Recuperation and Rest

Let's investigate a variety of tactics to use for the best outcomes now that we are aware of the justification for rest and recuperation.

1. Make sleep a priority. It's the cornerstone of recovery.

Perhaps the most important factor in healing is sleep. Your body goes into a state of repair and renewal when you sleep, which encourages muscular development and general healing.

- **Aim for 7-9 hours:** To encourage the best possible recovery, make an effort to get 7-9 hours of good sleep every night.

- **Establish a routine:** By going to bed and getting up at the same time every day to maintain a regular sleep schedule.

2. Active Rest Days: Coordinating Recovery and Movement

Complete rest days are important, but doing modest, low-intensity exercises on rest days can encourage blood flow and speed up recovery without adding to the body's stress.

- **Walking:** A brisk stroll is a great way to keep in shape without putting too much strain on your body.

- **Yoga:** Mild yoga sessions can improve relaxation, flexibility, and mobility.

3. Fueling Recovery with Food

- **A healthy diet:** This is essential for healing because it gives your body the resources it needs for growth and repair.
- **Protein Intake:** To aid with muscle recovery, consume enough protein.

Excellent options include lean meats, dairy products, eggs, and plant-based sources like beans and tofu.

- **Carbohydrates:** Refilling glycogen reserves with carbohydrates gives you energy for upcoming workouts. Choose fruits, veggies, and whole grains.

- **Hydration:** Maintain an appropriate level of hydration to promote cellular activity, blood flow, and nutrient delivery.

4. Stretching and foam rolling: reducing muscular tension

Stretching and foam rolling are crucial parts of rehabilitation that help reduce muscle tension and increase flexibility.

- **Foam Rolling:** To target tight muscles and loosen knots, roll the foam roller over them. Self-myofascial release is the name of this method.

- **Static Stretching:** Use static stretches to preserve joint range of motion and increase flexibility.

5. Self-Care with Massage: Promoting Recovery

Regular massages, whether performed by a licensed therapist or by self-care methods, can ease aching muscles, increase blood flow, and promote relaxation.

- **Self-Massage Equipment:** Invest in equipment to target certain muscle regions, such as massage sticks or percussion instruments.

- **Stress Reduction:** To aid with mental recuperation, incorporate stress-reduction practices such as mindfulness, deep breathing, and meditation into your daily routine.

6. Progressive Overload: An Equitable Strategy

Progressive overload is the practice of gradually raising your workout intensity over time. This strategy avoids overtraining while allowing for steady growth.

- **Listen to Your Body:** Look out for indicators of weariness, lingering aches, or a decline in performance. Your exercise volume and intensity should be adjusted accordingly.

7. Periodization: Intensity of Cycling

Periodization is the process of breaking up your training program into several stages of changing intensity. With this method, development is maximized and plateaus are avoided.

- **Microcycles:** Brief cycles that change in volume and intensity over the course of a week or two.
- **Mesocycles:** mid-term cycles with a typical duration of a few weeks to a few months and centered on certain training objectives.

- **Deloading weeks:** These weeks should be incorporated to allow for healing without hindering progress.

8. Cross-Training: Change Up Your Routine

Different forms of exercise, including swimming, cycling, or hiking, might modify the stimulation while resting particular muscle groups.

- **Active recovery:** select low-impact exercises that enhance joint mobility and circulation.

Supplements and Recuperation

While whole foods should be the cornerstone of your nutrition strategy, supplements can help heal and supplement your efforts. Some supplements to think about are:

- **Protein Powder:** A protein shake can help you satisfy your protein requirements when whole-food sources of protein are not available.

- **Creatine:** It has been demonstrated that taking creatine supplements increases strength, power, and muscular development.

- **Omega-3 Fatty Acids:** With their anti-inflammatory qualities, these fats can help maintain healthy joints.

- **BCAAs:** Branched-chain amino acids may limit the breakdown of muscles after hard exercise.

- **Multivitamins:** Make sure you're getting all the necessary vitamins and minerals to aid in recuperation.

Rest and recuperation are crucial components of a successful fitness journey; they are not decadent indulgences. By putting these tactics into practice, you not only avoid burnout and injury but also give your body the time and resources it needs to become stronger and more robust.

Keep in mind that growth involves both honoring your body's need for rest and pushing your limitations. Accept rest and recuperation as essential parts of your training regimen, and you'll see improvements in your performance, gains, and general wellbeing.

Chapter 7: Avoiding Plateaus and Overcoming Challenges

Starting a fitness journey is a commitment to your well-being and personal development. Whether you want to increase your power, lose weight, or have more endurance, the trip is characterized by thrilling advancement and sporadic setbacks.

Among these barriers, trials and plateaus pose as powerful foes that put your resolve and tenacity to the test. In this detailed book, we'll examine the causes of plateaus, analyze frequent obstacles, and provide you with practical tips for overcoming them so you can keep moving forward toward success.

Understanding Plateaus: A Progress Stagnation

Any fitness endeavor will inevitably experience plateaus, which are defined by a temporary stop in progress despite persistent effort. Any part of your fitness program, including strength increases and weight reduction, might experience these plateaus. They can be really aggravating since they appear to defy all of your effort and commitment.

The Reasons Behind Plateaus:

Your body is surprisingly good at adjusting to new difficulties. It becomes used to your training regimen over time, which leads to slower growth.

1. **Physiological Factors:** Age-related changes, hormonal changes, and genetic predispositions can all cause plateaus.

2. **Nutritional Unbalance:** Poor nutrition or inadequate calorie intake might impede fat reduction, muscle gain, and recuperation.

3. **Overtraining:** Pushing your body past its breaking point without enough rest can result in physical and emotional exhaustion, which can lead to plateaus.

Overcoming Obstacles: Techniques for Ongoing Improvement

1. Periodization: The Cycling Craft

Periodization is the process of breaking up your training program into sections, each with a particular emphasis and level of intensity. This strategy helps you overcome plateaus and keeps your body from adjusting to a particular regimen.

- **Microcycles:** Brief cycles with varied training conditions that typically last a week or two.

- **Mesocycles:** mid-length cycles (ranging from a few weeks to months) intended to focus on particular physical fitness objectives.

- **Deload Weeks:** Include lighter training weeks to give your body time to recuperate and adjust.

2. Progressive Overload: Gradually Increasing Intensity

The idea behind progressive overload is to gradually raise the intensity of your workouts. Increased repetitions, greater weight lifts, or changing other training factors can all be used to achieve this.

3. Exercise Variety: Keep it Dynamic

By changing exercises, rearranging routines, and adding fresh training methods, you can add variety to your workouts. This helps you make continual improvements by preventing your body from adjusting to repetitive stimuli.

4. Active Recovery: Rest's Function

Overtraining can frequently lead to plateaus. Active recuperation days, when you perform easy exercises like swimming, yoga, or walking, encourage blood flow and lessen weariness without taxing your muscles.

5. Nutritional Assessment: Promoting Growth

Examine your diet carefully to make sure you're giving your body the nutrients it needs for improvement and recuperation.

- **Protein Intake:** Consuming enough protein promotes muscle development and repair. Excellent choices include lean meats, dairy products, eggs, and plant-based foods like lentils.
- **Carbohydrate Balance:** Refueling glycogen reserves with carbohydrates gives athletes the energy they need for exercise and recuperation. Choose whole grains, fruits, and vegetables that are rich in complex carbs.

- **Enough water:** maintaining enough water is important for cellular activity, the movement of nutrients, and general health.

6. Mind-Muscle Connection: Concentrating

Your mind-muscle connection may be improved by mindful exercise participation, resulting in more efficient sessions and perhaps even breaking through plateaus.

7. Recovery Emphasis: Give Rest Priority

Rest is essential for muscle recuperation, development, and general growth. Try to get 7-9 hours of good sleep every night, and schedule rest days into your schedule.

8. Reconsider Objectives: Altering Viewpoints

To rekindle your desire and motivation, set new goals. These objectives may include particular accomplishments like lifting a certain amount of weight or finishing a predetermined number of reps.

9. The Strength of Positivity in Mental Resilience

Keep an optimistic outlook. Mentally taxing plateaus might occur, but keeping your attention on your accomplishments and picturing your intended results can support your perseverance.

10. Seek Professional Support: Expert Guidance

Consider getting advice from fitness experts or personal trainers if plateaus continue or obstacles appear insurmountable. Their knowledge can offer customized answers and modifications to help you get through obstacles.

Challenges and plateaus are a necessary part of any fitness journey. But they don't always mean failure. You may overcome plateaus and maintain your momentum by including periodization, increasing overload, diversity, and appropriate recuperation into your program.

Accept these tactics as a means of overcoming obstacles and as a constant reminder of your tenacity and commitment. Although progress may have its ups and downs, with perseverance, consistency, and the appropriate techniques, you will come out stronger, fitter, and more victorious than ever.

Chapter 8: Advanced Training Techniques

Using Advanced Training Methods, You Can Improve Your Fitness Level

You could find yourself looking for new challenges and opportunities to advance as your fitness adventure develops. Advanced training methods are useful in this situation.

These methods push the limits of conventional exercises, resulting in increased levels of strength, endurance, and general fitness. This thorough book will cover a variety of advanced training methods, their advantages, and how to incorporate them into your routine to increase your fitness.

Recognizing Advanced Training Methods

Advanced training methods are specific approaches intended to improve different fitness-related qualities. They are frequently employed to break progress plateaus, give new stimuli, and create diversity. These methods might be strenuous and demanding, but when used wisely, they can provide stunning results.

Utilizing Advanced Training Methods:

1. Efficiency in Action with Supersets and Compound Sets

Supersets entail executing two workouts consecutively without a break. By combining workouts that target the same muscle region, compound sets extend this idea. This technique promotes muscle endurance and growth by reducing rest periods while intensifying workouts.

2. Drop Sets: Exceeding Boundaries

Drop sets entail working out to failure, instantly lowering the weight, and then repeating the activity. By using this method, you exhaust your muscles' fibers and promote muscular development.

3. Gradual Intensity Pyramid Training

Pyramid training entails gradually changing the weight as you finish each set. This technique promotes adaptation by putting your muscles through a range of intensity degrees of stress.

4. Negative Reps: Exaggerated Accent

Negative repetitions concentrate on reducing the weight during the eccentric part of an exercise. Strength increases are facilitated by these repetitions, which focuses on muscular tension during the lengthening period.

5. Intense Breaks for Rest-Pause Training

Rest-pause training entails working through a set until failure, pausing for a while, and then continuing with more reps. This method optimizes metabolic stress and muscular activation.

6. Controlled Motion: Time Under Tension

TUT slows down the lifting and lowering stages and accentuates the length of each repetition. This method encourages muscular growth and enhances activation of muscle fibers.

7. Static Challenge: Isometric Holds

Isometric holds entail halting in the middle or at the finish of an exercise and holding it for a certain amount of time. This method improves muscle stamina and strength at particular joint angles.

8. Plyometrics: Powerful Explosion

Rapid and explosive actions, such jump squats or box jumps, are a part of plyometric workouts. These workouts enhance athletic ability and explosive power.

9. High-Intensity Interval Training: Increasing Cardiovascular Fitness

High-intensity interval training (HIIT) alternates between rest or low-intensity exercise segments. It increases metabolic rate, increases calorie burn, and enhances cardiovascular fitness.

10. Volume and Intensity in German Volume Training (GVT)

GVT is executing ten sets of ten repetitions with a moderately high weight for a single exercise. This high-volume method puts the muscles' fibers under stress and encourages hypertrophy.

11. Combining strength and power via complex training

Complex training involves combining strenuous resistance workouts with quick movements, such squats and box jumps. This method simultaneously increases strength and power.

12. CrossFit and functional training: a holistic approach to fitness

Functional training and CrossFit use a variety of workouts and apparatus to simulate real-life activities. These exercises improve coordination, strength, and general fitness.

The advantages of advanced training methods include:

Advanced methods make it possible for progressive overload, a concept essential for continuing growth. You may encourage development and adaptability by putting your heart and muscles through fresh challenges.

1. **Breaking Through a Plateau:** If you've reached a stop in your development, advanced tactics can give your body the jolt it needs to push through and reach new milestones.

2. **Time Efficiency:** Many advanced strategies are intended to make your exercises harder so you can do more in less time.

3. Challenges and variety for mental stimulation Maintain variety in your workouts to avoid mental boredom.

Safely Using Advanced Techniques:

Advanced procedures can provide amazing effects, but it's important to use prudence and the right technique while using them.

- **Gradual Progression:** To give your body time to adjust, introduce advanced methods gradually.

- Maintain appropriate form to minimize risks of injury and enhance rewards.

- **Recovery:** To avoid overtraining, make sure you have enough rest and recovery time in between tough sessions.

- **Professional Advice:** If you're unfamiliar with sophisticated procedures, think about speaking with a fitness expert to ensure a secure and efficient application.

The use of advanced training methods offers a dynamic and productive way to advance your fitness journey. Supersets, drop sets, pyramid training, and other exercises are just a few of the methods you may use to push your body to its limits and get unmatched results.

Always pursue difficult skills mindfully and seek assistance as needed, keeping in mind that safety and appropriate technique are crucial. You'll achieve new levels of strength, endurance, and general fitness as you include these strategies into your routine, which will inspire you to work harder and more resolutely toward your objectives.

Advanced Training Methods for Men: Physique Transformation, Power Gain, and Muscle Growth

Advanced training methods provide a dynamic way for men to improve their physiques, add muscle, and increase power as they continue on their fitness journey. These exercises stretch the limits of conventional workouts and inspire new heights of strength and performance by putting the body through novel challenges.

In this thorough book, we'll examine a variety of cutting-edge training methods designed especially for guys, emphasizing muscle growth, power improvement, and total physical change.

Unlocking the Potential for Hypertrophy in Muscle Building

For many men looking to build a strong and well-defined physique, hypertrophy—the process of muscle growth—is a significant objective. By encouraging muscle fiber recruitment and boosting growth, advanced approaches can elevate muscle building to a new level.

1. Cluster Sets for Hypertrophy: Rapid Reps

A set is divided into clusters of two to five repeats, with a short pause in between each cluster. By using this technique, you can lift heavier weights and still exert the same amount of force.

2. Pump and Growth with Blood Flow Restriction (BFR) Training

During low-weight, high-repetition exercises used in BFR training, blood flow to the muscles is restricted using resistance bands. This method induces metabolic stress that encourages the development of muscle and endurance.

3. Targeted Fatigue for Growth Using Myo-Reps

Myo-reps entail doing a set until it is nearly impossible, then taking a little break and executing further "mini-sets. By using this method, muscle fiber activation is maximized, encouraging hypertrophy.

4. The Triple Rep System

In 21s, you complete 7 partial reps in the bottom half of an exercise, 7 partial reps in the top half, and 7 full-range reps to finish. This method significantly increases the muscular pump and promotes development.

Increasing Strength: Activating Explosive Strength

Speedy force generation, or power, is necessary for activities like running, leaping, and explosive motions. Men can improve their power and explosive strength with the use of advanced training methods.

1. Explosive movements during plyometric exercise

Exercises called plyometrics feature quick, explosive motions like box jumps, clap push-ups, and medicine ball throws. These workouts increase explosiveness and power.

2. Technical Power Moves in the Olympic Lifts

Olympic lifts like the clean, jerk, and snatch require both a powerful explosion and exact technique. These exercises can improve your whole-body coordination and power.

3. Controlled explosiveness in ballistic training

Ballistic training entails doing explosive motions with weights below your maximum capacity. Exercises that train fast-twitch muscle fibers and increase power include medicine ball slams and kettlebell swings.

4. Depth Jumps: Training Jumps

Depth jumps entail falling from a height and then jumping as high as you can right after. This method improves vertical leaps and explosive power.

Changing Your Body: Creating a Chiseled and Lean Appearance

Men who want to gain muscle and lose fat might benefit from cutting-edge methods that combine the two to produce a sculpted image.

1. Circuit training: fusion of cardio and strength

With little respite in between exercises, circuit training includes executing a sequence of them. This method, which combines strength and aerobic components, burns calories while also gaining muscle.

2. Fat-Burning Intervals in High-Intensity Interval Training (HIIT)

Short bursts of intense exercise are interspersed with rest or low-intensity activity during HIIT. This method increases the metabolic rate and expedites fat reduction.

3. Combining strength and plyometric exercises

Complex training involves combining strenuous resistance workouts with quick movements such as squats and box jumps. This method encourages the growth of both power and strength.

4. The Quick and Effective Tabata Protocol

Tabata is a four-minute workout that consists of 20 seconds of intense activity followed by 10 seconds of rest. This strategy increases cardiovascular fitness while burning fat.

Men may remodel their bodies and increase muscular growth with the use of advanced training techniques. Men may go on a path of unmatched strength, power, and beauty by adopting techniques like cluster sets, BFR training, plyometrics, and circuit training.

Keep in mind that mastering these methods calls for endurance, reliability, and attention to appropriate posture. You'll redefine your fitness potential as you incorporate these strategies into your regimen and discover new realms of physical power.

Chapter 9: Safety and Injury Prevention: Protecting Your Fitness Journey

Starting a fitness journey is a commitment to your well-being and personal development. While there are many advantages, it is crucial to put safety and injury prevention first in order to make sure that your growth is both sustainable and injury-free.

Whether you're a novice or seasoned athlete, it's critical to comprehend injury prevention concepts and put safety measures in place. In-depth discussion of the significance of injury prevention, an examination of typical injury triggers, and recommendations for doable safety measures are all included in this thorough reference.

Injury Prevention's Importance: A Basis for Success

Injury prevention is an essential component of any successful fitness journey and goes beyond simple prudence. Why making injury avoidance a key priority is as follows:

1. Progress is ongoing: Injuries might interfere with your training schedule, causing setbacks and plateaus in your advancement.

2. Long-Term Well-Being: Making injury prevention a top priority promotes long-term fitness and health, enabling you to continue living an active lifestyle for years to come.

3. Cost savings: Preventing accidents helps you save medical expenses, out-of-pocket expenses for physical treatment, and probable time away from work.

Finding the Offenders: Common Sources of Injuries

You can take preventative action for injuries by being aware of their underlying causes. Typical reasons include

1. Poor Technique: Using the wrong form when exercising puts unneeded strain on the muscles and joints.

2. Overtraining: Overuse injuries can result from pushing your body over its limitations without enough rest.

3. Insufficient Warm-Up: By skipping warm-up activities, the risk of strains and sprains might be increased.

4. Unbalanced training: Injuries and physical imbalances can result from ignoring particular muscle groups or favoring one side of the body.

5. Rapid Progression: Overloading your body with too much weight, intensity, or volume can lead to injury.

6. Recovery Deficit Fatigue and higher injury risk might result from neglecting to prioritize rest and recovery.

Your Defense Against Setbacks: Injury Prevention and Safety Techniques

Maintaining proper technique and form is key when performing workouts. If necessary, get advice from fitness experts or personal trainers.

Gradual Progression: Increase weight, intensity, and volume gradually to give your body time to adjust.

1. Warm-Up and Cool-Down: To prepare your muscles and joints for exercise, set aside time for a dynamic warm-up before exercises and static stretching afterward.

2. Design a well-rounded exercise program that works all the major muscle groups and corrects any physical imbalances.

3. Rest and recovery: To give your body time to repair and renew, prioritize getting enough sleep, schedule rest days, and engage in active recovery.

4. Foods high in nutrients should be consumed, and you should drink enough water to assist muscular function and general recuperation.

5. Take Note of Your Body: Pay attention to any indicators of pain, weariness, or discomfort. Ignoring discomfort can make injuries worse.

6. Utilize a variety of workouts to minimize overuse injuries and improve general fitness through cross-training.

7. Wear proper footwear that offers enough support for the activities you choose.

8. Use a Spotter or Proper Equipment: To protect your safety when lifting big objects, use a spotter or the appropriate tools.

9. Include Mobility Work: To increase joint range of motion and avoid stiffness, regularly perform mobility exercises.

10. Consult experts: If you're unsure about your form or technique, consider working with a licensed physical therapist or personal trainer.

11. Keep Up-to-Date: Become knowledgeable about appropriate practices, workout adaptations, and methods for avoiding injuries.

12. Modify as Necessary: If a workout causes pain or discomfort, adapt it or swap it out for a more secure option.

Your fitness path should focus on injury avoidance and safety. You may lower your chance of setbacks and lay the groundwork for long-lasting improvement by comprehending the typical causes of injuries and putting tactics like good technique, moderate progression, balanced training, and adequate recuperation into practice.

Keep in mind that caring for your body is essential for both reaching your fitness objectives and preserving your general well-being. As an investment in your long-term health, embrace the concepts of injury prevention and allow them direct you on a fulfilling and injury-free exercise path.

Conclusion

Your Path to Strength, Transformation, and Resilience, in Summary

Congratulations on finishing this thorough overview of strength training, cutting-edge methods, injury prevention, and general fitness. We've looked at the nuances of building a robust, long-lasting body while cultivating a solid foundation of health and wellbeing throughout this book. Let's consider the main lessons learned from this experience and the lasting effects it may have on your life as you end this chapter.

Strength that Goes Beyond the Body

Strength training is a way to develop mental toughness, discipline, and self-awareness in addition to building muscle. The length of your potential and the extent of your resiliency are revealed on this voyage. You'll see how your body changes as you accept the difficulties and successes of each activity, as well as how your mind develops and becomes more resilient.

Goal-setting and plan-design:

Setting definite, attainable objectives and developing a unique plan to achieve them are the cornerstones of a successful fitness journey. You've given yourself the tools to travel the road ahead with purpose and direction by establishing your goals and creating a plan.

Innovative Methods for Improved Performance:

The options are endless in the field of sophisticated training methods. These methods provide you with the keys to unlocking new levels of strength and capacity, from adding muscle and increasing power to shaping your body. Keep in mind that mastering these skills calls for persistence, patience, and a commitment to safety and appropriate form.

Putting safety and injury prevention first

Injury avoidance and safety are not only measures in your quest for physical perfection; they are pillars on which your advancement is built. You've created a strong fortress against setbacks by using injury prevention techniques, enabling your trip to go on without interruption.

Acknowledging the Journey

Your passion for bettering yourself, for health, and for vitality is demonstrated through your fitness journey. Whether you lift a bigger weight, complete a difficult workout, or simply feel more energized and confident in your daily life, it's a path that celebrates every success.

Progress and Persistence:

Keep in mind that growth is not always linear; setbacks and plateaus are regular traveling companions. Utilize your inner fortitude in these situations, put the techniques you've learned to use, and have faith in the course of events. Every obstacle is a chance to show your everlasting resolve, and every failure is an opportunity for a return.

Discover your future:

Think about the future you are creating as you proceed, equipped with the information and insight you have gained from this book. Imagine yourself as someone who embodies fortitude, resiliency, and vigor in all facets of their life. Your fitness journey will pay off in your behaviors, demeanor, and general well-being, whether you're at the gym, at work, or spending time with loved ones.

A permanent commitment

Your road to improving your general fitness, strength training, and advanced methods is not limited to a few weeks, months, or even years. It's a dedication to living a healthy, fulfilling life and always improving oneself. As you move through the phases of life, keep learning, growing, and adapting while constantly embracing the chances and difficulties that come your way.

Final Thoughts

As you begin the road ahead, keep in mind that you have the power to mold your future, shape your body, and develop a resilient and strong attitude. Your path is special, and it's worth goes well beyond the material world. Accept the knowledge gained, the accomplishments made, and the development made.

We appreciate you choosing this book to be your travel companion while you pursue health. May your journey be one of success, development, and unwavering faith in your unbounded potential. Here's to a life full of fortitude, change, and the unrelenting pursuit of excellence.